The Pain Free Workbook With Yoga Secrets

Use the Ancient Wisdom of Yoga To Stop Chronic Pain

KEN HEPTIG

Ken Heptig

For information, submit a request: Goalyoga.com/connect

For bulk rate book discounts visit: http://goalyoga.com/book-bundles/

Publisher: IT CIRCUS LLC

Charlotte, NC USA

Cover design by Anna Thompson

The author of this book does not dispense medical advice or prescribe any technique as a form of treatment for any physical, emotional, or medical problems without the advice of a physician, directly or indirectly. Readers should consult their own doctors or other qualified health professionals regarding the treatment of any medical conditions. No liability is assumed for losses or damages due to the information provided. You are responsible for your own choices, actions, and results.

ALSO BY KEN HEPTIG

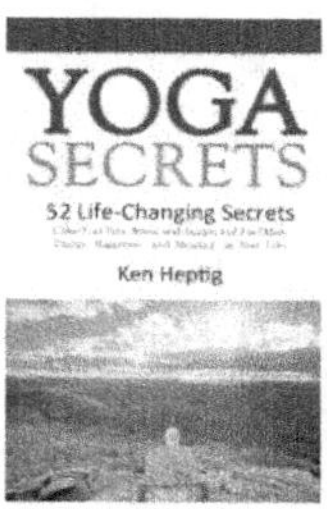

Yoga Secrets: 52 Life-Changing Secrets
Calm Your Pain, Stress, and Anxiety and Find More
Energy, Happiness, and Meaning in Your Life.

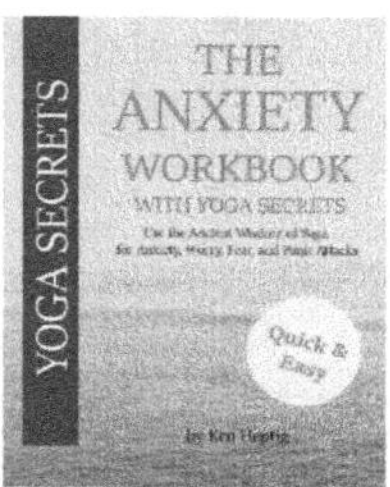

The Anxiety Workbook With Yoga Secrets
Use the Ancient Wisdom of Yoga for Relief from Anxiety, Worry, Fear,
and Panic Attacks.

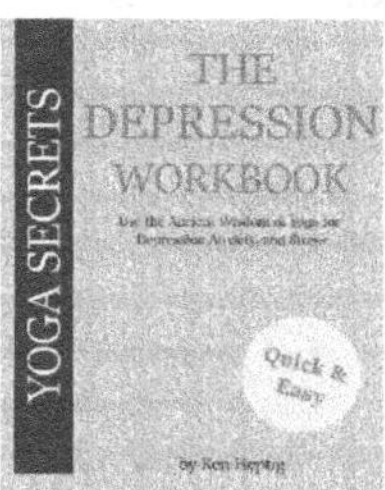

The Depression Workbook With Yoga Secrets
Use the Ancient Wisdom of Yoga for Relief from Depression and Anxiety.

Contents

1 PAIN

A panic attack goes from zero to 100 in an instant.

Goal – Live Pain Free

One of my students purchased a 400-page workbook on self-help. If I had to work through 400 pages on pain, it would cause my pain to have pain. I might decide that I would be better off to do nothing and just live with my current level of pain.

There has to be a better way. I have been practicing yoga for two decades and knew yoga could offer a different solution. I have spent over a decade weaving the ancient wisdom of yoga into my classes while my students practiced yoga. This required me to refine the secrets until they were quick and easy. I tested the secrets in thousands of classes. This inspired me to create a workbook using the quick and easy lessons from yoga secrets. They are so easy my students could learn them while practicing yoga.

The yoga classes I taught while refining the secrets varied from advanced power hot to relaxing restorative yoga. At first, it was very awkward teaching the secrets. It was not working. I could not find books or articles that could help. My physical yoga practice taught me you could become better at most things with practice. I kept refining the simplicity and clarity in each lesson until they were quick and easy. Then one day I realized I was connecting my student's physical world with their spiritual experience.

The ancient wisdom of yoga has gifted you amazing insight into the workings of the human mind and body. One of these amazing gifts is clarity. In ancient times, Tibetan Monks discovered that when things get messy in your life you need a clear mind to find your way. The problem is that when your life gets messy your mind also gets messy. Their solution was to practice having a clear mind when your life is not messy. This helps you find a clear mind when your life gets messy. Yes, the richest part of yoga is the spiritual and it requires practice. Tibetan monks still use the single word clear-seeing.

Types of Pain

Pain is the most common reason people visit their doctor. Chronic pain usually fits into one of two categories. Nociceptive pain occurs when there is damage to body tissue and is usually an aching, sharp, or throbbing pain. Neuropathic pain happens when there is actual nerve damage and it is a burning, heavy, numbness sensation along the path of the affected nerve.

Most common location of chronic pain

- Back pain
- Headache pain
- Joint pain

Nociceptive Pain - Specific pain receptors are stimulated.
- Somatic
- Arthritis
- Back pain
- Fibromyalgia
- Headache including migraines
- Joint pain
- Muscular ischemia
- Neck pain
- Pelvic pain

Visceral pain - felt in the organs of the major body cavities
- Endometriosis in women
- Irritable bowel syndrome
- Prostate pain
- Bladder pain

Non-nociceptive pain - caused by the nerves
- Pinched or impinged nerve
- Sciatica
- Peripheral neuropathy
- Shingles
- Neuroma
- Multiple sclerosis

Sympathetic
- Complex regional pain syndrome type I and II
- Sympathetically maintained pain

Other forms of chronic pain
- Psychogenic pain - no obvious physical cause
- Anxiety
- Depression
- Somatoform

Idiopathic pain - no known cause

Causes and Sources of Chronic Pain

Common causes of chronic pain

- Arthritis
- Back problems
- Cancer pain
- Depression
- Endometriosis in women
- Fibromyalgia
- Headaches including migraines
- Infections
- Injuries
- Joint pain
- Nerve damage and neuropathy
- Psychogenic pain - no obvious physical cause

Common sources of chronic pain

- Joint pain
- Abdominal pain
- Arthritis pain
- Back pain
- Cancer pain
- Chest pain
- Fibromyalgia
- Headache pain
- Neck pain
- Nerve damage pain
- Osteoarthritis
- Pelvic pain
- Postsurgical pain
- Post-trauma pain

Chronic Back Pain

Common locations of chronic back pain

- Lower back
- Middle back
- Upper back

Common causes of chronic back pain
- Arthritis - discs in the spine lose the ability to absorb shock, which causes bones to rub together
- Bulging or slipped disc - a soft disc between the vertebrae that extends out over the edge
- Osteoporosis - brittle, weak bones can break and create compression fractures
- Pinched nerve - your nerve presses up against the bone
- Pregnancy - extra weight puts a strain on the back
- Referred pain - intense pain in another part of the body causes you pain in your low back or groin
- Sciatica – sciatic nerve runs from your lower back to the back of each leg, when pinched it can cause lower back pain and a sharp pain in one or both legs

Common sources of chronic back pain
- Compression fractures
- Slipped or bulging discs
- Soft tissue damage
- Spinal stenosis
- Structural deformities
- Traumatic fractures

Things that increase the risk of chronic back pain
- Ageing
- Heredity
- Job - lifting, pushing, pulling, or twisting your spine and sitting at a desk for long periods of time with poor posture
- Other diseases - certain types of arthritis and cancer
- Overweight
- Poor physical fitness
- Smoking - can reduce the nutrients to the disks in your back

Chronic Headaches

Tension headaches are the most common form of headache. It usually feels like a dull band of pain, sensed across both sides of the head.

Common types of headaches
- Cluster headaches
- Eye strain headaches
- Headaches from illness or medications
- Migraines
- Muscle tension headaches

Factors contributing to tension headaches
- Poor sleep
- Bright lights
- Fatigue
- Poor posture
- Stress

Chronic Joint Pain

The most common location of chronic joint pain in order
- Knee pain
- Shoulder pain
- Hip pain

Common types of chronic joint pain
- Osteoarthritis - wear and tear on joints over time
- Rheumatoid arthritis - causes swelling in the joint spaces
- Repetitive strain injury – usually in larger joints like the knee or shoulder

Symptoms of chronic joint pain
- Joint redness
- Joint swelling
- Joint tenderness
- Joint warmth
- Limping
- Locking of the joint
- Loss of the range of motion of the joint
- Stiffness
- Weakness

2 MENTAL HEALTH

Often the term mental health refers to mental illness. Although related, they are different emotional states.

Mental health is an emotional state of well-being about your abilities to cope with the normal stress of daily life. Mental illness includes all diagnosable mental disorders or health conditions that cover alterations in mood, thinking, and behavior. It includes your social, emotional, and psychological well-being. The ability you have to become a member and contribute to your community. It affects how you feel, think, and behave. It determines how you handle stress, your relationships, and the decisions you make. Studies show that positive mental health improves overall mental health.

Factors Contributing to Mental Health
- Biological factors like genes and brain chemistry
- Life experiences like trauma or abuse

Ways to Calm Your Anxiety
- Connecting with others
- Getting enough sleep
- Helping others
- Learning coping techniques
- Physical exercise
- Positive attitude

Warning Signs of Mental Health
- Arguing more with friends and friends
- Avoiding people and usual activities
- Changes in appetite and weight
- Feeling helpless, hopeless or numb
- Feeling more confused, angry, worried, forgetful, or scared
- Hearing voices or believing things that are not true
- Inability to handle daily tasks for your kids, work or school
- Increase in drinking, smoking, or drugs
- Lack of energy
- Obsessive thoughts and memories
- Severe mood swings
- Sleeping too much or not enough
- Thinking of harming yourself or others
- Unexplained aches and pains

Cognitive Distortions

"The primary cause of unhappiness is never the situation, but your thoughts about it."

—Eckhart Tolle

Cognitive distortions are a distorted or biased way of thinking about yourself and the world. These thinking patterns can reinforce your negative thoughts. They can bolster the effects of mental disorders, especially in anxiety and depression. They can interfere with the way you perceive events.

Cognitive distortions offer specific ways you distort your thinking. The way you feel affects how you think. These distorted thoughts can increase negative emotions creating a negative outlook on the world.

Cognitive distortions that can increase your level of anxiety, stress, and worry

- All-or-nothing thinking   Seeing things in only black-or-white with no middle ground
- Always being right   Always trying to prove your opinions and actions are correct
- Blaming   Holding other people responsible for your pain
- Expecting bad outcomes   Expecting the worst-case to happen
- Control fallacies   Feeling controlled
- Diminishing the positive   Believing positive events do not matter
- Emotional reasoning   Believing the way you feel reflects reality
- Fallacy of change   Expecting other people will change to suit you
- Fallacy of fairness   Feeling resentful because you think you know what is fair
- Filtering   Focusing on the negatives and filtering out all the positives
- Heaven's reward fallacy   Expecting sacrifice and self-denial to pay in the afterlife
- Jumping to conclusions   Creating negative interpretations without evidence
- Labeling   Beliefs based on mistakes and shortcomings
- Overgeneralization   Basing things on only one negative experience
- Hypersensitive   Taking things on a person level
- Strict limits   Strict beliefs about what you should and should not do

3 PAIN TOLERANCE

"That's the thing about pain, it demands to be felt."

—John Green

Pain is usually unavoidable when you stub your toe, twist an ankle, or cut your finger. You immediately feel your pain, although it only feels bad for as long as you allow it to feel bad. Your brain produces pain, which is why a lot of your pain is in your head.

Factors That Affect Pain Tolerance

Insomnia
Having trouble sleeping can reduce your tolerance to pain. One study found that participants with insomnia more than once a week, had significantly lower pain tolerance than without insomnia.

Depression
Depression can affect pain. It can manifest itself as physical pain. Based on one study, people who suffered from depression had significantly more frequent, intense, and unpleasant pain complaints when compared to healthy people.

Drugs
Certain drugs may cause or more pain instead of relieving it. Opioids like oxycontin and vicodin can do more harm than good. You can become more tolerant and dependent when using a drug.

Genes
Genes help determine your sensitivity to pain. The gene bh4 increases pain sensitivity. Blocking bh4 makes you less sensitive to pain and reduces your risk for chronic pain.

Gender
A study found females have a lower pain threshold than males. One reason is the female body releases fewer natural painkillers (beta-endorphins) than the male body. Another possible reason is females have evolved sensory mechanisms that make them more in tune to changes across all senses, including feeling pain.

Your brain
The wiring in your brain may influence your tolerance of pain. One study finds a correlation between your sensitivity to pain and the thickness of the cortex in the brain. Other studies reveal that less gray matter in the brain can indicate a higher level of pain sensitivity.

Exercise levels
The amount of exercise you get affects your level of pain tolerance. After exercising, healthy people had a higher threshold for pain. Although, people already suffering from chronic pain experienced mixed results, depending on the pain conditions.

Hair color

Research suggests that being a redhead can make you more sensitive to pain. Redheads require more anesthesia. One reason may be a mutation in a gene called mc1r that causes red hair. The mc1r gene receptors are in the same family as pain receptors.

Stress

Stress affects your body's ability to manage pain because of the physical and emotional effects it has on the body. It can also contribute to anxiety and depression that can cause lower pain tolerance.

Change Your Pain Tolerance

Studies suggest that you can change your pain tolerance by changing your perception of pain. Look at the pain that you feel as nothing more than information. Tell your body that this pain information is good pain or tell your body to simply ignore this information and not react to it. If you tell yourself the pain is not good for you, then your body will harden and your muscles will contract leading to even greater pain. Think about how athletes learn to embrace the pain or push through the pain.

Trick your brain into not feeling any pain

Pain is generally unavoidable. When you stub your toe, cut your finger, or break your leg pain happens instantly. Sometimes it lasts for a long time, but pain feels bad only as long you allow it. Pain is in your head.

Overload yourself with positivity to lessen the hurt

It might seem absurd, when you are suffering from pain, but positive thoughts and emotions can overcome the bad feelings of pain.

Distraction

Distract your brain from feeling the pain. Distract your mind by laughing, using visualization, and relaxation techniques.

Practice mindful meditation

Meditation is the art of sitting still and letting the mind run wild. With only a few minutes of stillness, you can relax and unwind. You can also retrain your brain to feel less pain.

Laughter and humor

Laughter and humor can help distract you from your pain. It also provides a great endorphin release. It is better to be laughing with other people or in a social setting. You are more likely to laugh when you are in the presence of others. One study, published in Ethology, claims you are 30 times more likely to laugh with others than by yourself.

4 DESCRIBING PHYSICAL PAIN

"If you can sit with your pain, listen to your pain and respect

your pain, in time you will move through your pain."

—Bryant McGil

One way to describe pain is to use a scale of 1 to 10 with 10 being the highest level. Anyone can describe your pain. Although, you are the only one who can feel your pain and you need to decide how to describe your own pain.

Questions to Help You Describe Your Pain

- Increasing and decreasing factors - What makes the pain better or worse?
- Character of the pain - Is it sharp, dull, throbbing, or burning?
- Environment - Where does the pain occur, at work, home, or somewhere else?
- Other symptoms - Is it weakness, nausea, numbness, or something else?
- Severity - Use a 0 to 10 scale from no pain to the worst pain ever.
- Duration - How long does the pain last and is it constant or intermittent?

Common Types of Pain

- Achy pain - a part of your body feels achy resulting in continuous but not strong pain

- Acute pain - strong and sharp pain

- Agonizing pain - very painful

- Angry pain – a bad wound or cut that is red and painful

- Bad pain - a part of your body that is not working well and causes you pain

- Burning pain - a feeling that part of your body is touching something hot

- Chapped pain - skin or lips being dry and painful often from cold weather

- Chronic pain - serious pain lasting a long time

- Crippling pain - a lot of pain or other health problems

- Dull pain - weak pain but continues for a long time

- Excruciating pain - extreme physical pain

- Gnawing pain - causing you continuous pain

- Heavy pain - a part of your body feels heavy and uncomfortable making it hard to move

- Inflamed pain – a part of your body is inflamed, swollen, red, and painful due to an injury or infection

- Irritated pain - red or swollen and painful

- Itchy pain - an unpleasant feeling on your skin making you want to scratch it

- Raging pain - very serious, painful, or strong

- Raw pain - your skin is raw and sore

- Severe pain - injury or illness that is serious and unpleasant

- Sharp pain - sudden and severe pain

- Sore pain - uncomfortable, usually from infection, injury, or too much exercise

- Stabbing pain - a sudden, strong pain

- Stiff pain - a part of your body is stiff and you feel pain in your muscles restricting your movement

- Stinging pain - hitting you hard

- Tender pain - part of your body is tender from injury and is painful when you touch it

- Tight pain - your chest or another part of your body feels tight as if being squeezed

- Torturous pain - extreme physical pain

- Unendurable pain - too unpleasant or painful to bear

- Vice-like pain - holding or squeezing feeling resulting in pain

- Violent pain - painful and difficult to control

5 WORKBOOK GOALS

- Live pain free forever.
- Learn and practice specific techniques to calm your pain.
- Learn breathing techniques to calm your emotions, soften your body, and calm your pain.
- Create personal mantras to change how you think about pain.
- Turn negative self-talk into positive self-talk creating a powerful force in your life.
- Find and replace bad habits with good habits.

Simplicity and Clarity

Yoga has taught me to strive for clarity in everything I do. This workbook embraces quick and easy based on simplicity and clarity.

The Pain Free Workbook with Yoga Secrets follows three easy steps.

Three Easy Steps
1. Understanding a concept
2. Learning a technique
3. Practicing until it becomes a habit

Perhaps number three is increasing your anxiety and physical pain. Relax and breathe. Would you rather practice something 4 pages long or 400 pages long? This does not mean you have to keep practicing it forever. You need to keep practicing the technique until it feels like a subconscious reaction and becomes a habit.

In your effort to understand your world, you continuously break things down into smaller pieces. When you strive for simplicity and clarity, it moves you to increasingly smaller pieces of your world. Your mind can more easily understand ideas if you organize, compare, and create levels. As you try to create greater levels of clarity, you increase complexity and loose simplicity. Remember your goal is to live pain free forever.

Many of you find it hard to make changes that will stick. Most people fail when trying to make permanent changes because they stop trying too early. People also fail when they do not practice implementing what they have learned in their daily lives. Throughout this workbook, you will practice ways to inspire change and find freedom from anxiety. Each of the exercises provides an introduction, benefits, techniques, and practice. Take the tools you learn in this workbook and apply them to your daily life. Change requires constant attention and effort. As you keep practicing the techniques, notice the progress you are making towards your goals.

Simple Works

> "Simplicity is the ultimate sophistication."
>
> —Leonardo da Vinci

Simple solutions face two mental obstacles.

I am not wrong.
Most of you hate being wrong. Finding out you missed something simple hurts your ego and makes you feel stupid.

My belief system is not wrong.
Simple challenges your belief system. It challenges the belief system of your tribe. Sometimes it challenges your career, your job, and invalidates what you believe and have been working for your adult life. These are strong reasons you reject simple solutions. Many of you refuse to change your belief systems.

Belief:	**Hard work**	**= Better results**	**= Better solutions**
Misbelief:	**Simple solutions**	**= Less work**	**= Worse solutions**
Misbelief:	**Complex solutions**	**= More work**	**= Better solutions**
Truth:	**Simple solutions often**	**= More work**	**= Better solutions**

Remember your goal is to live pain free forever. Consider the end of the next two paths.

Path 1 – More and More Clarity Forever

Reading, understanding, and practicing your 400-page book, to stop your pain, could create ever more clarity and sophistication. It has you spending more time obsessing and focusing on different types of pain. It compares and contrasts different theories about pain. You are spending large amounts of time reinforcing that you have a problem with pain. You now have more time, work, and emotions invested in your pain. Maybe you discover your pain is now a much bigger and more dominant part of your life. Does this seem like what you are trying to avoid? Those doctor visits and pain pills, with harmful side effects, for the rest of your life.

Path 2 – More Simplicity, Mindfulness, and Enjoy Life

Traveling down the path of more simplicity minimizes the time you spend reinforcing your pain, making it a smaller more manageable part of your life. This gives you more time to enjoy your new pain free life.

6 YOGA

I recommend that you start a physical practice of yoga. It should help quicken and deepen your personal lifetime transformation.

Starting Your Yoga Practice

You should at least try several beginner classes. This will help you learn the name of the poses, alignment, and use of blocks and straps. It will also increase your comfort and confidence when taking your first non-beginner class. A good yoga foundation can increase your chances of making yoga an ongoing practice in your new personal lifetime transformation.

When you start your yoga journey, keep an open heart and an open mind. Keep going to class and do not stop too soon. Listen to your teacher to learn the poses and alignment. It is fine to look around to make sure you are doing the correct pose. However, do not compare yourself to your classmates and be overly judgmental. This is not a competition. Work on enjoying your practice.

Before starting
- Consider starting with a beginner class
- Be honest about your current level of fitness
- Decide on what level of yoga class you want to take
- Shop around for prices and new student special deals

Finding yoga classes
- Yoga studio
- YMCA
- Fitness club or gym
- Search online for keywords free, cheap, or donation yoga classes
- Do not get talked into a contract
- Look for a one or five class pass
- Try several different places

Other options
- Buy a DVD
- Online yoga programs
- Private yoga lessons
- Yoga classes on your television

Things to do
- Get to know your classmates
- Learn to use blocks and a strap
- Stay until the end of class

Things to know

- Be kind to your body and to yourself.
- Keep an open heart about you experience.
- Let go of attachments and practice.
- Others are not watching you; they are focusing on how they look, the alignment of their pose, and deepening their practice.

Physical Benefits of Yoga

Improves

- All-round fitness
- Athletic performance
- Balance
- Breathing ability of your lungs
- Cardio and circulatory health
- Cartilage and joint strength
- Flexibility
- Immune system functionality
- Posture
- Respiration and vitality
- Sleep

Increases

- Blood flow
- Bone strength
- Energy
- Heart rate
- Muscle strength

Decreases

- Blood pressure
- Blood sugar
- Digestive problems
- Muscle tension
- Problems with allergies and viruses
- Spine problems

Other
- Maintains your nervous system
- Regulates your adrenal glands
- Relaxes your system
- Supports your connective tissue
- Uses sounds to soothe your sinuses

Emotional Benefits of Yoga

Improves
- Ability to stay drug free
- Aliveness in the present moment
- Awareness for transformation
- Body's healing in your mind's eye
- Calmness
- Concentration
- Happiness
- Healthy lifestyle
- Inner peace
- Intuition
- Memory
- Mind-body connection
- Mood
- Positive outlook on life
- Relationships
- Self-acceptance
- Self-control
- Self-esteem
- Social skills

Decreases
- Anxiety
- Depression
- Fear
- Hostility
- Pain
- Stress
- Worry

7 THE ANCIENT WISDOM

Yoga Secrets

> The longest journey is the journey inward.

Yoga does not focus on your goal or destination. Instead, the focus of yoga is to help you on your journey through life. Yoga is a method to help avoid and manage threats and obstacles during your journey. When you follow this yoga method it can help lower your anxiety and help you flow through life with ease.

In *The Pain Free Workbook with Yoga Secrets*, the reference to yoga refers to the non-physical philosophy or the spiritual side of yoga. This part of yoga can help you handle your thoughts and sensations when events happen that elicit your response. It can help you stay mindful and overcome obstacles and challenges. You can learn specific yoga techniques to help manage your thoughts, sensations, threats, obstacles, and challenges during your journey.

Yoga Secrets is an easy way to learn and enjoy the ancient wisdom of yoga. Yoga Secrets is a term I used in my book *Yoga Secrets: 52 Life-Changing Secrets*. The book follows the same path as the ancient wisdom from The Yoga Sutras Eight Limbs of Yoga by Patanjali. The ancient wisdom is about two thousand years old and offers guidance on how to live a meaningful and purposeful life.

When I started my yoga practice, my teachers used phrases like "Be mindful," "Set an intention," and, "Stay present." Rarely did they explain the meaning of these terms. When they did, it was vague and confusing. When other students heard the phrases, they flashed big smiles of joy. I was a beginner with little knowledge of yoga. Although my human senses could not detect what was happening, my mind still created an explanation. That explanation was wrong and created more misbelief in my mind. I believed the students with the big smiles were telling the world they truly understood and had found enlightenment. I practice what I learn, and "joy" and "happiness" were among the concepts in yoga. My happiness for my fellow students who had found enlightenment was sincere. Although, I still found these phrases confusing and it continued to be depressing.

I became more confused which continued to increase my anxiety. I wondered why I am still confused while the other students easily understood. It was time to put my ego aside, I asked the enlightened students to explain the meaning of the phrases. I told them I did not understand the phrases used in class. They responded with silence, and then they looked confused. After a long pause they responded with, "Well, uh…you know, I'm not really sure what they mean."

I decided the phrases used in class were to generate good feeling and entice students back to class. With that in mind, I created the term "placebo phrase" to show they were empty phrases to generate good feeling. After that, it was easy to smile.

As time went by, these placebo phrases became more empty and meaningless. They kept increasing my confusion and anxiety. After extensive research and reading, I felt I understood the meaning of many of the life-changing lessons of yoga. My next step brought back the confusion and anxiety when I tried teaching the lessons to my yoga students in a fun, easy, and clear way.

The challenge was making the secrets so easy and clear I could teach them while students practiced yoga. This required constant testing and refining over 10 years and thousands of yoga classes. Yoga teaches you to seek the truth in life. This usually requires questioning and changing your beliefs as you seek that truth.

The Eight Limbs of Yoga

"Mastery of yoga is really measured by how it influences our day-to-day living, how it enhances our relationships, how it promotes clarity and peace of mind."

—T.K.V. Desikachar

The Yoga Sutras of Patanjali, created sometime from between 100 to 300 CE, had people practicing them long before the text. The Eight Limbs of Yoga are in the second chapter of The Yoga Sutras. Patanjali is the author or compiler of *The Yoga Sutras,* and many call him "the father of yoga." Although, perhaps the writing came from multiple contributing authors over several generations.

Around 3,500 years ago, yoga was a spiritual, meditative practice. It did not include postures or physical practice. Hatha Yoga changed this in the tenth century and included physical postures, pranayama breath control, and spiritual intention. Yogis found it difficult sitting for a long time during meditation as they tried to connect with the spiritual world. Practicing physical yoga poses made it easier to meditate, focus, and move into stillness. The physical practice of yoga became a portal to the spiritual world.

To study yoga in ancient times, you had to move and go live with your teacher. Imagine people doing that today!

The Eight Limbs of Yoga is a systematic method of levels like the levels referenced in this workbook when explaining the "Anxiety Severity Scale". A yogi goes through the levels from limb one to limb eight. Notice that only one of the eight limbs is about asana or the physical practice of yoga.

The last or eighth limb is Samadhi. It means enlightenment or union with the divine. During the Eight Limbs, you remove your identity and obstacles. As you practice the first two limbs, yamas and niyamas, you work through a process called attainment, fruits, or acquisition. The attainments uncover things already there. The first five rungs or limbs sharpen your razor or attention for discrimination. You then use this sharpened razor in the last three limbs concentration, meditation, and Samadhi to peel away your layers of habit and misbelief and find your true self.

Limb #8 Samadhi (Enlightenment)

The eighth or final limb of yoga is samadhi. You work through the first seven limbs, in order, before achieving the eighth or final limb of yoga. Patanjali describes this stage as transcendence of the self through meditation, you move beyond time, form, and space. Samadhi is the ultimate stage in yoga, where you find a supreme consciousness.

In the early state of samadhi, you lose self-consciousness or your sense of I. The process of meditation and the object of meditation become one.

Samadhi is a series of states and experiences. The Yoga Sutras of Patanjali describe various types of samadhi you need to pass through on your way to enlightenment. The highest stage of illumination is dharma megha samadhi. This liberates you from all the limitations of the body and mind.

During samadhi, you achieve discriminative enlightenment, where you use viveka, razor-like attention to divide the seer and the seen.

The Yoga Sutras Eight Limbs of Yoga

#	Limb	Description
1	Yama	universal morality (values)
2	Niyama	personal observances (laws)
3	Asanas	body postures
4	Pranayama	breathing, control of prana:
5	Pratyahara	control of the senses
6	Dharana	concentration, perception, awareness
7	Dhyana	devotion, meditation on the divine, being keenly aware without focus
8	Samadhi	union with the divine

Limb #1 Yama - Universal Morality (Values)

The first limb is the yamas. They are moral constraints to focus on how you behave and conduct yourself in your life. They guide you to restrain behaviors that come from grasping, aversion, hatred, and delusion. Yamas suggest avoiding violence, lying, stealing, greed, and wasting energy.

The five yamas	Description
Ahimsa	nonviolence, kindness
Satya	Truthfulness
Asteya	non-stealing
Brahmacharya	moderation, continence
Aparigraha	generosity, non-covetousness

Limb #2 Niyama - Personal Observances (Laws)

The five niyamas refer to self-discipline and spiritual practices. They include the wellbeing of yourself and others. Rather than telling you right or wrong, the niyamas are rules for you to follow. They do not mention heaven or hell. Niyamas suggest, rather, that you avoid behaviors that produce suffering and embrace those that lead to happiness. Niyamas let you create harmony within you and with your external world, without telling you what to do. That is for you to decide.

Benefits occur when you remove identity and obstacles. Patanjali describes this process as attainment, fruits, or acquisition. This attainment comes from uncovering what is already there.

The five niyamas	Description
Saucha	cleanliness, purity
Samtosa	Contentment
Tapas	heat; spiritual austerities
Svadhyaya	study of the scriptures and oneself
Isvara Pranidhana	surrender to god

8 NON-REACTION: THE POWER TO CHANGE AN EVENT

If you cannot control your thoughts, the world will control them for you.

Your mind has evolved to seek the negative. During evolution, you faced many predators and obstacles that could end your life. This might have created a fight-or-flight reflex, which increases your heart rate and causes your breath to become irregular. Many of those predators and obstacles are no longer a threat to your survival, yet you still treat minor threats as if they are.

Learn to keep minor events from triggering your fight-or-flight reflex. When a non-urgent event elicits a response, you can practice nonreaction. You pause and you do not react to the event. This gives you time to decide if you even want to react to the event. The need to react to an argument or perceived obligation is often insignificant or based on your own misbelief.

With nonreaction, you discover you are not your thoughts and sensations. You are that space between thoughts and sensations, which yoga calls your true self.

A subtle difference exists between awareness of a thought and thinking a thought. Awareness of a thought is a texture or a light, distant feeling. Thinking a thought elicits tension in your body like contracting a muscle, an increase in your heart rate, or an irregular breath.

One way of practicing nonreaction is by becoming an observer and noticing your thoughts. When you pause and do not react to an event, it gives you time to catch and notice your thoughts. That quiet time between thoughts and sensations, allows you to observe your thoughts and notice your habits. Practicing nonreaction creates a pause in your actions and emotions. This gives you time to decide how to react or perhaps to not react at all. It helps keep your emotions, habits, and misbelief from deciding for you. Nonreaction keeps the world from controlling your life through your emotions.

Learning to Watch Your Thoughts

Learn to watch your thoughts. It is like watching the clouds come and go as they float through the sky. You notice the clouds, but you do not attach yourself to the clouds. You only observe the clouds as they come and go. When you practice nonreaction, you observe without instantly reacting. Nonreaction helps you find freedom from the world that controls you through your emotions.

Nonreaction allows you to change your thoughts and improve your life. It takes practice and mindfulness to stay in the present moment. When you slow your thoughts and sensations, it helps you with stress, concentration, anxiety, clarity, happiness, and freedom. Practice can make this easier so it will feel more natural and like an automatic reflex.

Observing events allows you to act as a bystander so you can notice how your habits and misbelief control you when things happen. You can see how you live your life. When you stay in the present moment you do not control your thoughts, you just keep your thoughts, habits, and misbelief from controlling your life. Nonreaction provides you with an opportunity to calm your mind, concentrate, and move into stillness. It gives you an opportunity to notice and change your habits and misbelief.

Your reaction to an event has the power to change the event. Find that space between your thoughts and sensations, your true self. When you find that quiet space, you will find stillness. In stillness, you can find freedom from your anxiety.

9 PHYSICAL EXERCISE

If you only exercise when you feel good, how will you ever exercise

often enough to feel good all the time?

Fitness means being able to do physical activity and having the energy to function at as high a level as possible. You can improve your health by getting even a lit bit more fit. Start slowly and gradually, and then increase your intensity. If you have any type of health condition, you should talk with your doctor before starting.

It is important to avoid inactivity. Any amount of physical activity is better than inactivity and has health benefits.

The Center for Disease Control recommends, for a healthy adult:
   2.5 hours per week of moderate-intensity aerobic physical activity like brisk walking or tennis.
   Or
   1.25 hours per week of vigorous-intensity aerobic physical activity like jogging or swimming laps.

Anything good for your heart, is usually great for your brain. Aerobic exercise is great for your body and brain. It improves brain function and can act as a "first aid kit" on damaged brain cells. Physical activity can improve your cognitive function during your life regardless of your age.

Three-Legged Stool

Yoga believes everything in the universe connects with everything else in the universe. To live a healthy life you must have a yin (passive) and yang (vigorous) balance. The yin and yang act to complement one another creating balance and harmony. You need the same balance for the interrelationship between a clear mind, a strong body, and an enlightened spirit.

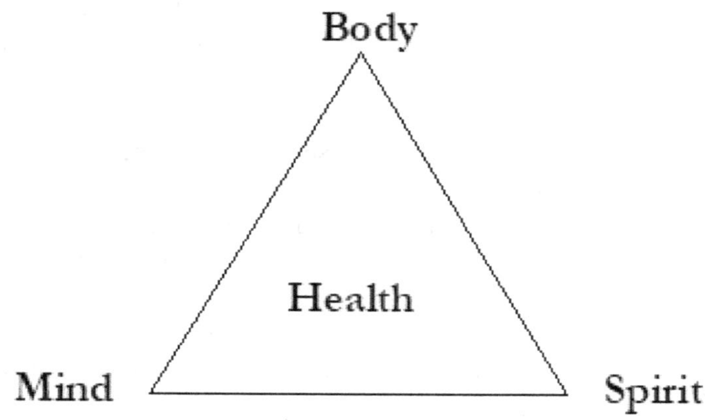

Benefits of Physical Exercise

Pain is temporary and will subside while quitting makes it last forever.

Exercise can be a very effective treatment for physical pain. Although, without the side effects of pain medication. When you maintain your exercise schedule, it can help keep you pain free from a previous pain or from new pain.

Exercise relieves stress and tension that can increase physical pain. It releases endorphins in your brain increasing your energy and making you feel good. It also distracts you from your physical pain, anxiety, and negative thinking.

Instant Benefits of Exercise

The moment you start your exercise the benefits of exercise begin. Changes start in seconds with an increase in your heart rate and blood pumping to your muscles. You start to burn calories and get an almost instant mood boost.

Increases

- Ability to control addiction
- Brainpower
- Capacity to function
- Chance of longevity
- Creativity
- Energy
- Happy chemicals
- Memory
- Mental health and mood
- Productivity
- Relaxation
- Self-confidence
- Sleeping comfort
- Strength of bones and muscles
- Weight control ability

Lowers

- Anxiety
- Cardiovascular disease
- Cognitive decline
- Risk of certain cancers
- Stress
- Type 2 diabetes

10 TECHNIQUES

"Yoga provides us tools and techniques to lead a stress-free and a tension-free life."

—Sri Sri Ravi Shanka

A technique is a method of doing a task or performing something. Yoga uses very specific techniques to perform a wide range of specific tasks. The ancient wisdom of yoga left you a wide variety of very specific breathing techniques.

1 Breathing
You will explore breath awareness, breathing to calm your emotions, and Ujjayi Pranayama Breathing. With proper technique, breathing can soothe the nervous system, calm the mind, relax the muscles, soften the body, lower blood pressure, lower the heart rate, and calm physical pain. You will practice breath awareness and breathing techniques.

2 Self-talk
Your message to yourself matters. Your body hears every thought you think and word you speak. It reacts to everything you tell yourself. Clarity in your words creates clarity in your life.

You will use motor imagery, positive versus negative self-talk, positive thinking, clarity, and Mantras to help you change negative self-talk into positive self-talk.

3 Mantras
Yoga believes the words you think or say out loud produce a physical vibration. Repetition of these words and the physical vibration can change how you view your world.

4 Personal Mantras
The words that work with my belief system are very different from the words you should use for your belief system. For mantras to work you must feel comfortable and believe in the words you use.

5 Habit Shifting
Bad habits keep you from accomplishing goals and from fully living your life. Those that break a bad habit often replace it with a different habit. Bad habits waste your prana or life force. Use your life force energy to focus on the important things in your life.

You will practice shifting a habit from bad to good regardless of the habit you are trying to break. To shift a habit you will use triggers, awareness, patterns, learning to unlearn, and not giving up too early.

11 WAYS TO MANAGE PAIN

"Find a place inside where there's joy, and that will burn out the pain."

—Joseph Campbell

Learn how to change the way you think about your pain, stress, and anxiety. To feel pain, you have to see yourself and your pain as separate from one another. Then when pain occurs, you try to run away from your pain. You soon realize that running away from your pain does not work and causes suffering.

Instead of trying to run from your pain, try to get inside your pain. Give your sensation of pain your undivided attention so that nothing else receives any of your attention. This leaves you no space for wanting to stop your undivided attention. Then you can decide if this sensation leans towards pain or pleasure.

To keep from running away from your pain, try staying in the present moment. Look for interesting things you can find using your senses like sights, smells, touch, tastes, and sounds. Identify anything you can sense in the present moment. Noticing as many sensory inputs as possible can dilute your pain and turn it into just one of many sensations.

Immediate Pain Treatment

- Acupuncture
- Controlled breathing
- Do something creative
- Distraction
- Epsom salt bath
- Exercise to produce endorphins
- Food fantasies - Shifts your focus away from pain.
- Hypnosis
- Imagery - Relaxes the body, mind, and distracts you from pain.
- Laughing
- Listen to music
- Mantras
- Massage
- Meditation
- Positive thinking
- Present moment
- Pressure points
- Simplify your sensations
- Visualization
- Writing
- Yoga

Long Term Pain Treatment
- Cut stress in your life
- Do not smoke
- Drink less alcohol
- Eat healthy
- Get enough sleep
- Herbal remedies - can reduce inflammation that can increase pain
- Join a support group on chronic pain
- Keep in touch with friends and family
- Learn biofeedback

Visualization Techniques for Pain
- Age progression and regression - Project yourself forward or backward in time to when you were pain-free. Now focus on this good feeling to help lessen your pain.

- Dissociation - In your mind focus on separating your painful body part from the rest of your body. Try to visualize body and mind as separate.

- Happy imagery – Identify a place in the past where you felt pain free, calm, and relaxed. Focus on this happy feeling.

- Sensory splitting - Divide your sensation of pain into separate parts. What looked like a permanent solid block are many different sensations that are always changing. See chapter 15 on Mantras for more examples.
    - Burning, hot, warm, cool, cold
    - Intense, moderate, mild, weak
    - Sharp, blunt, dull, soft

- Transfer a sensation - Use your mind to create an altered sensation, such as heat or cold, in a non-painful hand. Place that hand over the painful area. Imagine transferring this pleasant, altered sensation of heat or cold into the painful area. This distracts your mind away from focusing on the source of your pain.

- Transfer your focus - Switch your focus to a part of your body that is pain-free. Relax as you focus on your pain-free sensation and allow it to become your main sensation.

- Two point approach - Identify a point number one that could be the center of your pain. Choose point number two, a place on your body that does not hurt. It could even be a place outside your body such as where you find peace and relaxation. Hold the first and second point in your mind. Visualize and focus on both points simultaneously. Now go do something else. Upon your return, have you eliminated or notably softened your pain?

12 USING YOGA TO MANAGE PAIN

The Bhagavad Gita states that the man to whom pleasure and pain are alike, and who is wise becomes eligible for immortality. If you can learn to relax your pain during physical exercise, it should become much easier to relax your pain when you are not exercising.

When you are experiencing pain during your practice of yoga, try balancing the opposite feelings of effort and surrender. This can help relieve the strain of your physical task and lessen your pain. Try the below techniques I recommend during my yoga class.

Ways to Soften Pain While Practicing Yoga

- Breathing - Learn to breathe using a steady and calm breath throughout your entire day. It is important to do this even when you are pain free. For more information read chapter 13 about breathing with a steady and calm breath.

- Leave your ego at the door. The practice of yoga offers healing energy which requires little strain and effort. You have nothing to prove and you do not have to compete with others in your class.

- Listen to your body. The sensations that occur in your body tell you what is happening in your body. You can tell if you are experiencing good pain or bad pain. Your body tells how far to push. Work towards softening into your practice and letting go of habits and patterns in your body that hold tension. Try to find a level of ultimate sweetness during your practice. This occurs when your pose becomes effortless.

- Practice contentment - Ease up on yourself and stay within your limits. When you push yourself to a level of exhaustion, you increase your chance of injury. Try practicing with a more relaxed mind and body. It may allow you to go further in your physical practice and open a path to more growth. Try to find the ultimate sweetness in your practice as you play with the delicate balance of effort and surrender.

- Soften and release your lines of energy - The lines of energy in your body can release heat you might interpret as pain. This energy creates a sensation that can feel exhilarating and challenging or it can be short and sharp. You have a choice in deciding how you interpret the feelings you have during your sensations.

- Soften your facial muscles and the tension in your jaw - Try to get rid of the frown, exhaustion, or struggle you are wearing on your face. Replace it with a little smile. I get my yoga students to soften the expressions on their faces by telling them to transition to the next pose with a fake smile. I also tell them to transition to the next pose with only half of a smile. Later in the class, I ask them to add the other half of a smile to even out their smile. Both techniques soon turn into a real smile.

13 BREATHING

Breathing Introduction

Change how you breathe, to change how you see.

Pain can keep you from living the life you desire and deserve. The problem is you cannot live without feeling pain. The good news is you really can learn to manage your pain, using simple techniques, so you can live pain free. This allows you to more fully experience and enjoy your life in the present moment.

Before you begin, you need to understand why you might find yourself trapped with chronic pain. Your mind has evolved to seek the negative including pain. During evolution, you faced many predators and obstacles that could end your life. This might have created a fight-or-flight reflex, which increases your heart rate and causes your breath to become shallow and irregular. Pain can warn you about problems and help you stay alive. Many of these are no longer a threat to your survival, yet you still treat them as if they are a serious threat. This causes your brain to release sensations that feel like pain.

Learn to practice non-reaction. When an event elicits a response, which is not urgent, simply pause and do not react. This gives you time to decide how you want to react or not react. This becomes easier with practice and by staying mindful. For more information visit chapter 8 on Non-Reaction: The Power To Change An Event.

Breathing techniques can help you calm and manage your pain. You can learn to control your emotions and reflexes using breathing techniques. This changes the way your subconscious views yourself. Practice can make you better at most things. Keep practicing these exercises until they become habits. These exercises can help you find freedom from your pain.

Yoga does not teach you to pretend that things are not happening around you. Events will always happen around you. Yoga does not teach you to lie to yourself. This would create confusion and an unhealthy journey through life. Instead, yoga teaches you to seek the truth and manage what is happening around you so you can flow through life with ease.

Breathing in yoga is your Prana or life force connection. Pranayama breathing is the control of your life force through your breath. Pranayama is the measuring, controlling, and directing of your breath. When you join the inhale with the exhale, you find perfect relaxation and balance in all your body activities and functions.

Proper breathing gives more oxygen to your mind and to your body. Pranayama breathing helps you enjoy more happiness, weight loss, energy, and a longer life. Yoga can teach you how to integrate your breathing, mind, and emotions. This can help you keep your emotions, thoughts, and habits from controlling your life. In yoga, you do not control your thoughts; you just keep your thoughts from controlling you.

When you slow down and pause, you are rising above the noise of your thoughts and sensations. This allows you quiet time to observe your thoughts and sensations. When you pause before reacting, you find freedom to become the person you wish to be rather than allow your past habits to control your life.

Breathing to Calm Emotions

"Its not stress that kills us, it is our reaction to it."

—Hans Selye

The power and benefits of yoga breathing over the central nervous system, has sparked the interest of scientists and doctors for years. You can divide your nervous system into two modes: sympathetic (fight or flight) and parasympathetic (rest and digest). The sympathetic "fight or flight" phenomenon developed as a survival mechanism in ancient times. The sympathetic activates the adrenal medulla gland, which then releases hormones into the bloodstream. These hormones cause the body to speed up, tense up, and become more alert. The parasympathetic system kicks in even when no immediate threat or danger is present. Long periods of relaxation lets the body return to balance and recover as the immune and digestion systems take priority.

Although you become more alert when you activate your sympathetic nervous system, experts found that it takes a huge toll on your body. This evolved as a way to protect you from real physical dangers like dangerous animals or people. You can also trigger your sympathetic nervous system with other stressful situations like work deadlines, arguments, or too much anxiety.

At first, researchers believed you could not control this automatic switch between the systems even if there was no true physical danger. In the 1970s, Dr. Herbert Benson published his book "The Relaxation Response". In it, he describes breathing techniques used by eastern health practitioners and yogis for centuries. The book argues that one could trigger the parasympathetic nervous system to kick in and counter the fight or flight response to daily stresses by controlling one's breath. Since then, multiple studies have expanded upon and proven his theory that breathing techniques can override your body's automatic switch to the "fight or flight" mode.

You can learn to invoke the opposite reflex, the relaxation response. To do this you need to use a proper breathing technique to calm this reflex. Continuous practice of breathing for your relaxation response can help you change your fight-or-flight reflex and keep it from responding as often during your day. I find it amazing that it took until the 1970's for the western culture to recognize and claim, as their discovery, something Yogis have known for centuries.

Learning breath-control techniques, and staying mindful of your breath, allows you to gain control over your respiratory system and your life. Be mindful of how your breath, mind, and emotions weave together. When breathing with a steady and calm breath you can lower your heart rate, slow the activity in your brain, calm your emotions, soften your body, relax your muscles, and calm your pain. You strengthen your respiratory system, soothe your nervous system, and lower your external cravings.

Breathing can make a healthy person sick or a sick person healthy. It cleanses your lungs, oxygenates your blood, and purifies your nerves. It calms the mind of negative emotions and stress. Your breathing reveals your inner feelings and emotions. It connects what you know with what you feel. Steady and calm breathing can calm physical pain, mental stress, depression, anxiety, worry, fear, and panic. It can improve your health and increase your happiness. Exhale the bad and inhale the good.

Calming your desires and cravings gives you freedom from emotions, habits, and misbelief. Freedom from your emotions helps your mind move into stillness giving it space for concentration.

Breathing Exercises

> When you own your breath, nobody can steal your peace.

Instructions:

During these three exercises on breathing, you will practice being aware of your natural breath. You will then learn and practice a steady and calm breathing technique and an Ujjayi pranayama breathing technique.

Exercise 13.1 - Breath Awareness

Using this breathing technique, you focus your complete attention on one point, which is your breath.

1. Sit or lie down in a comfortable and quiet place. Relax and close your eyes. Place your left hand just below your navel and your right hand over your heart. Breathe in and out using a steady and a calm breath. All breathing is through your nose while keeping your lips sealed.

2. Try to tune into the natural flow of your breath. Do not try to control your breath in any way. Simply observe your breath.

3. Notice how you feel as you inhale. What happens in your body? Where do you feel your breath go?

4. How do you feel at the crest of each inhale? Do you notice any changes in your body during the pause before you exhale?

5. Notice how you feel when you exhale. Where does the point of exhalation start? Is the pace of your inhale different from exhale?

6. What do you notice in the pause after your exhale, when you are empty of breath? Is this pause different from the pause after you inhale?

7. Learn to notice your breath as it flows in and out of your body. Notice the small variations taking place in the flow of your breath. Notice whether your breathing feels comfortable or uncomfortable. Change your posture. Notice any sensation of breath in your new position. Notice any sighing or unusual breaths. Do not become anxious or feel you need to react. Simply observe your sensations. You are not your thoughts and sensations. You are that space between thought and sensation. Yoga calls this space your true self.

Steady and Calm Breathing

All life starts and ends with our breath.

Pranayama yoga breathing can increase energy, cut stress, improve mental clarity, and improve physical health. Although, all breaths differ in the effect and benefits they have on your body and your mind.

Most of you breathe from your chest that creates shallow breathing. This signals your brain that you have a problem and your brain responds by creating stress. When you breathe from your abdomen, it boosts respiration, increases the oxygen going to your brain, and signals to your brain that all is well.

Breathe with a steady and calm breath and make your exhales longer than your inhales. This replicates the body's natural breathing when resting and fools the body and brain into being more relaxed. This method of breathing triggers a change in your nervous system from sympathetic mode the fight or flight mode, to parasympathetic the rest and digest mode.

Exercise 13.2 - Breathing with a Steady and Calm Breath

Instructions:

Sit in a comfortable seated position where you will not have interruptions. Inhale through your nose for a count of 4, then exhale through your nose for a count of 6. Count your breaths using your fingers. Each count can be about 1 second long. With practice, you should be able to lengthen your number of inhales and exhales.

There are three important ingredients.
1. Make your exhale longer then the inhale
2. Breathe only through your nose for both inhales and exhales.
3. Practice the exercise and do not just read about it.

Practice your breathing using one of the below rhythms or create your own rhythm.
- Inhale 3, exhale 5
- Inhale 4, exhale 6
- Inhale 6, exhale 9
- Inhale 4, exhale 8
- Inhale 5, exhale 10
- Inhale 4, hold the breath for 4, exhale 6
- Inhale 4, hold the breath for 2, exhale 6

Set a timer and do this exercise for at least 3-5 minutes. Repeat daily or as often as you can until breathing with a steady and calm breath becomes a habit.

Ujjayi Pranayama Breathing

The translation for Ujjayi (pronounced oo-jai) is "victorious breath". Another name used is the "oceanic breath". Yogis have used Ujjayi breathing for thousands of years. You can improve how you feel by regulating the length, air volume, and sound of your inhales and exhales.

It is important to relax during Ujjayi breathing. Ujjayi breathing naturally lengthens your breath. Too much effort can cause a grating sound. To produce the pleasing ocean sound requires a delicate balance of not too little or too much effort.

All inhales and exhales are through your nose with your lips sealed. This helps to create a resistance to air from your breath. Nostril breathing helps you to support a steady, calm breath.

Your breathing should be smooth and steady. It should be continuous and uninterrupted cycles of inhales and exhales. To make the Ujjayi sound, seal your lips and take an inhalation through your nose that is slightly deeper than normal. Constrict the muscles in the back of your throat as you slowly exhale through your nose. Similar to the constriction you make when speaking in a whisper or if breathing through a thin straw.

Inhaling with a gentle and calm breath and exhaling against this resistance creates a steady and soothing sound. It should sound like the sound of ocean waves rolling in and out.

Notice if the sound between the inhales and exhales is the same. You can observe the quality of your Ujjayi breath by listening to its sound. Notice if your breathing feels strained, irregular, or forced.

Your breathing should feel energizing and relaxing. In the Yoga Sutra, Patanjali suggests that the breath should be both dirga (long) and suksma (smooth).

You can use specific breathing rhythms and techniques that can help your body, mind, and emotions.

Exercise 13.3 - Ujjayi Pranayama Breathing

Instructions:

1. Sit in a comfortable position.
2. Close your eyes and place your right hand over your heart and your left hand just below your navel.
3. As you inhale, feel how your belly expands. Take several natural, deep inhales and exhales.
4. Inhale and exhale through your mouth as if you were trying to fog up a mirror making a "HAAAAH" sound. Making noise is a part of this technique.
5. Seal your lips and take an inhalation through your nose that is slightly deeper than normal. Exhale slowly through your nose while constricting the muscles in the back of your throat.
6. Try to create the same sound and sensation while inhaling and exhaling.
7. Have fun playing with your Ujjayi Breathing by taking deeper breaths and pausing before exhaling.

Benefits of Ujjayi Pranayama Breathing

"Learn how to exhale, the inhale will take care of itself."

—Carla Melucci Ardito

Ujjayi breathing can soothe the nervous system, calm the mind, relax the muscles, soften the body, slow down the heart rate, lower blood pressure, and soften pain. When you focus on your breathing, you can calm the feelings of agitation. The fluctuations of your mind slow down and let you observe and not constantly react to your emotions. You can calm your pain with the steady and calm rhythmic nature of your Ujjayi breath.

You cannot have intense physical pain and perform Ujjayi breathing at the same time. It is about being able to change the way you feel by not letting your emotions control your life.

Calm

- Calms feelings of irritation and frustration
- Calms the mind and body
- A feeling of present and aware
- Calms pain
- Relieves tension

Heat and energy

- Builds energy
- Builds internal body heat
- Encourages the free flow of prana (life force)
- Instills endurance
- Regulates internal body heat

Focus

- Diminishes distractions
- Improves concentration

Balance and regulate

- Balances the cardio respiratory system
- Detoxifies the mind and body
- Maintains a constant rhythm while practicing yoga
- Increases the amount of oxygen in the blood
- Lessens pain from headaches
- Regulates blood pressure
- Relief of sinus pressure
- Strengthens the nervous and digestive systems

14 SELF-TALK

Self-Talk Introduction

"The most important decision we make is whether we

believe we live in a friendly or hostile universe."

—Albert Einstein

Here is Einstein's explanation of the above quote. If we decide the universe is an unfriendly place, we will create bigger walls to keep out the unfriendliness and may isolate or destroy ourselves. If the universe is neither friendly nor unfriendly, then we are victims of the random toss of the dice, and our lives have no real purpose or meaning. If we decide the universe is a friendly place, we will use technology and science to understand that universe. It is a simple principle: You get what you give.

If you suffer from chronic anxiety, you may see the world as a hostile universe or more dangerous than it actually is. You may think things will turn out poorly or treat negative thought as if it were fact. Cognitive distortions are pessimistic and irrational attitudes not based on reality. It is a misbelief and a habit causing you to react instantly to your emotions.

You hold internal conversations as you go about your daily life. Psychologists have named one of the most important forms as "Self-Talk". You give opinions and evaluations on what you are doing as you are doing it. When upbeat and self-validating, the results can boost your productivity and self-esteem. Negative self-talk can cripple your emotions. Saying nice things to yourself can boost your mood. Most people are unaware of the power of self-talk.

Neurologists have been exploring this concept for the past century. In 1911, for example, Dr. Henry Head and Dr. Gordon Morgan Holmes published a series of papers on a study they did on the mind-body connection. In the study, they used a style of hats that were very popular during that time. Fashionable women during the early 20th century were wearing large hats with giant feathers at the top. Holmes and Head noticed that women who often wore these big hats walked through doors, they always ducked even if they were not wearing the hat. Besides being funny, the study concluded that the subjects "mental self" was wearing the hat, even if their physical self was not. There are similar studies where patients with eating disorders turn to the side or try to "squeeze" through spaces in which they have plenty of room.

Although neuroscientists are still trying to understand how this works, it shows how your internal view of yourself affects how you function in the external world. You need a very specific sense of yourself to understand how to move and function. This allows you to walk and not bump into things, or reach out your hand to pick up a coffee cup without grasping for air.

Your message to yourself matters. Your body hears every thought you think and word you speak. It reacts to everything you tell yourself. If your message is unclear, you create stress and frustration for yourself and for others. You can change how you view reality by changing negative words to positive words. For example, you can soften your words and change "I feel pain" to "I feel discomfort." You can change "I am angry" to "I am curious."

You become what you think. A clear, positive message creates clear, positive thoughts. This can help you make better choices and enjoy a healthier and happier journey through life.

Motor Imagery

"All that we are is the result of what we have thought."

—Buddha

Other research includes what neurologists call "motor imagery". Findings on this internal sense of oneself shows you use the same neurological networks to both imagine movement and for actual movement. When you practice visualizing or imagining a movement, it can have the same effect on your brain as practicing it in the physical world. This can also lead to similar improvements in performance. Likewise, practicing positive thoughts and words can improve your overall self-esteem, silence your inner critic, and improve the reality of the world in which you live.

Positive Thinking

"Watch your thoughts; they become words.

Watch your words; they become actions.

Watch your actions; they become habits.

Watch your habits; they become character.

Watch your character; for it becomes your destiny."

—Upanishads, 800 to 500 BCE

Positive thinking does not mean you ignore or pretend that uncomfortable or painful situations do not exist. Your body listens to every thought you think and every word you speak. Positive thinking means you approach uncomfortable situations in a more positive and productive way. You stay mindful that you can manage these unpleasant situations. When you practice optimistic thinking, the best will happen, not the worst.

Positive thinking often starts with self-talk. Self-talk is the continuous stream of unspoken thoughts that run through your head. These thoughts can be positive or negative. Your self-talk comes from logic and reason. Other self-talk comes from habits or misbeliefs you get from others or misguided explanations you have created in your own mind. You can develop layers of misbeliefs that can be difficult to uncover in your search for your true self.

If you live with negative self-talk, your outlook towards the universe is more pessimistic and you are more likely to keep others out of your life. If you live with self-talk that is positive, you are more likely optimistic. You are more open to the world and you practice positive thinking. Research suggests that positive self-talk creates positive thinking, optimism, improved health, and a richer feeling of happiness.

A clear, positive attitude helps you create clear, positive thoughts. Use positive thinking with your new ability to manage your emotions and keep your emotions from controlling your life. Change how you see and find a new world.

Benefits of Positive Self-talk

"If you don't like something, change it. If you can't

change it, change the way that you think about it."

—Mary Engelbreit

Yoga believes the words you think or say out loud produce a physical vibration. Repetition of these words and the physical vibration changes how you view your world.

Repeating specific words can help you distract your mind from negative thoughts and physical pain. It can help you focus on a positive life. The Sanskrit word "mantra" means "instrument for thinking." The method is to repeat mantras when you relax, meditate, or any time you have available.

Benefits of positive thinking:

- ✓ Achieve goals
- ✓ Better athletes
- ✓ Higher coping skills
- ✓ Better organized thoughts
- ✓ Improved physical well-being
- ✓ Improves psychological well-being
- ✓ Greater resistance to the common cold
- ✓ Happier 9 to 5 working time
- ✓ Healthier
- ✓ Improves recovery
- ✓ Increases Confidence
- ✓ Less anxiety
- ✓ Less depression
- ✓ Longer life span
- ✓ More job offers and promotions
- ✓ Reduces anger
- ✓ Relives stress

Self-Talk - Moving from Negative to Positive

"I hear, and I forget. I see, and I remember. I do, and I understand."

—Confucius

Mantras for positive thinking

Exercise 14.1 - Selecting Positive Mantras

An article by Harvard Health Publications tells us that pain is depressing, and depression causes and intensifies pain. People with depression are three times more likely to develop chronic pain then the average person. This shows a strong link between the mind-body connection. Positive self-talk can make us more positive so naturally negative self-talk can make us more negative.

Use the below mantras to move from negative to positive self-talk.
    1 - Identify and place a check mark next to the positive mantras that work for you.
    2 - Practice saying your selected mantras out loud until they become a part of your belief system.

Present Tense Mantras
__ I am capable.
__ I know who I am and I am enough.
__ I will be present in all that I do.
__ I choose to think thoughts that serve me well.
__ I will reach for a better feeling.
__ I share my happiness with those around me.
__ My body is my vehicle in life; I will fill it with goodness.
__ I feel energetic and alive.
__ My life is unfolding beautifully.
__ I am confident.
__ I always observe before reacting.
__ I know with time and effort I can achieve.
__ I love challenges and the things I learn by overcoming them.
__ Each step on my path is taking me to where I want to be.

Practice speaking to yourself in the first person "I am capable" and speaking in the third person "Michelle is capable".

15 MANTRAS FOR PHYSICAL PAIN

Exercise 15-1 - Selecting Present, Future, and Natural Mantras
1 - In the list below, identify and place a check mark next to the mantras that work for you.
2 - Repeat the mantras you selected out loud until they become a part of your belief system.

Present Tense Mantras
__ I am pain free
__ I am not controlled by my pain
__ I am peaceful even when life is messy
__ I am relaxed
__ I easily release tension in my mind and body
__ I find it easy to relax
__ I focus on the future and not the past
__ My body is healthy and pain free
__ My mind is always calm

Future Tense Mantras
__ I am finding it easier to control my pain
__ I am always becoming more relaxed
__ I am always feeling less pain
__ I am finding it easier to not let life get me down
__ I am finding it easier to think positive
__ I will become pain free
__ I will find time to relax my mind each day
__ I will let go of the past
__ Positive thinking is beginning to help my pain

Natural Mantras
__ Being pain free is who I am
__ Controlling my pain is easy for me
__ Controlling my pain is effortless for me
__ I can control my body with my mind
__ I find it easy to release stress
__ I stay positive and pain free when things get messy
__ My body is always naturally relaxed
__ My mind is naturally calm and relaxed
__ Thinking positive is something I naturally do

16 CREATING PERSONAL MANTRAS

"Pain is always emotional. Fear and depression keep

constant company with chronic hurting."

—Siri Hustvedt

Belief Systems and Using Words that Work

The words that work with my belief system are very different from the words you should use for your belief system. For mantras to work you must feel comfortable and believe in the words you use.

When I train and certify yoga teachers, a 200-hour yoga certification, I use a 2-step process. First, I give them the exact words to use so they can learn how to teach a yoga class. As the students become comfortable teaching, they learn to teach using their own words. This makes them more confident, sincere, and successful when teaching yoga. Using your own words will make you more successful in your journey to become pain free.

Exercise 16.1 - Mantras for Specific Feelings of Pain

Instructions:

Use the below mantras for specific feelings of pain. You will also have the opportunity to create personalized mantras that focus on your specific feelings of pain while using your own words.

    1 - Identify and place a check mark next to the mantras that work for you.

    2 - Practice saying your selected mantras out loud until they become a part of your belief system.

____ My aching pain is disappearing
____ My burning pain is cooling
____ My dull pain is unimportant
____ My hot pain feels warm
____ My intense pain feels milder
____ My nagging pain is unfeeling
____ My sharp pain feels blunt
____ My shooting pain feels weak
____ My stabbing pain feels dull
____ My throbbing pain feels shallow

Exercise 16.2 - Creating Mantras for Specific Pain with Your Own Words.

Keep using the wording in the mantras, from Exercise 15.1, if they work for you. If the wording does not work, you should create your own mantras using your own words.

Identify and place a check mark next to the terms below that describe your pain.

Common terms used to describe pain
__ Aching
__ Burning
__ Dull
__ Hot
__ Intense
__ Nagging
__ Sharp
__ Shooting
__ Stabbing
__ Throbbing

From the words you selected above, identify and circle words in the below table you can use to shift how you think about your pain. If the above words do not accurately describe your pain, then visit chapter 4 about describing your pain. Use any of the words below that can lessen your pain.

Remember that your body hears every word you speak and every thought you think. When you shift the words you use, your mind can shift how your body feels your pain. The goal is to use words you believe can move you closer to a pain free life.

Aching	Burning	Dull	Hot	Intense
Blunt	Cool	Boring	Calm	Disappearing
Dull	Dull	Calm	Cool	Moderate
Mental	Soft	Flat	Mild	Slow
Shallow	Unfeeling	Gentle	Soothing	Tolerable
Tolerable	Unimportant	Low-Key	Unfeeling	Unimportant

Nagging	Sharp	Shooting	Stabbing	Throbbing
Boring	Flat	Blunt	Blunt	Disappearing
Gentle	Low	Calm	Flat	Occasional
Infrequent	Moderate	Mild	Smooth	Shallow
Low	Soft	Occasional	Unimportant	Slow
Stupid	Tolerable	Weak	Weak	Smooth

Exercise 16.3 - Creating Personal Mantras in Present Tense

Select a term you identified in chapter 15 that describes your pain.	Select a present tense mantra you identified in chapter 15.	Create a mantra using the term that describes your pain.
Example 1 • Intense	• I am peaceful even when life is messy.	• I am peaceful even when I feel intense pain.
1		
Example 2 • Throbbing	• I am not controlled by my pain.	• I am not controlled by my throbbing pain.
2		
Example 3 • Sharp	• I easily release tension in my mind and body.	• I easily release tension in my mind and body when I feel a sharp pain.
3		

Exercise 16.4 - Creating Personal Mantras in Future Tense

Select a term you identified in chapter 15 that describes your pain.	Select a future tense mantra you identified in chapter 15.	Create a mantra using the term that describes your pain.
Example 1 • Aching	• I will become pain free..	• I will become free of my aching pain.
1		
Example 2 • Burning	• I am finding it easier to control my pain.	• I am finding it easier to control my burning pain.
2		
Example 3 • Shooting	• I am always feeling less pain.	• I am always feeling less shooting pain.
3		

Exercise 16.5 - Creating Personal Natural Mantras

Select a term you identified in chapter 15 that describes your pain.	Select one of the natural mantras you identified in chapter 15.	Create a mantra using the term that describes your pain.
Example 1 • Intense	• I can control my body with my mind.	• I can control my intense pain with my mind.
1		
Example 2 • Dull	• Controlling my pain is effortless for me.	• Controlling my dull pain is effortless for me.
2		
Example 3 • Hot	• Being free of my pain is who I am.	• Being free of my hot pain is who I am.
3		

17 HABITS THAT AFFECT PHYSICAL PAIN

Diet
- Not eating enough vegetables
- Not getting enough calcium and vitamin D
- Poor eater

Exercise
- Being sedentary
- Bike seat not properly adjusted
- Lifting incorrectly
- Neglecting strength training
- Not exercising
- Not practicing yoga
- Not stretching
- Too many crunch exercises

Habits
- Cracking your knuckles
- Holding a grudge
- Ignoring pain
- Poor posture
- Relying on the wrong muscles
- Smoking and tobacco use
- Watching too much TV

Life Style
- Being overweight or obese
- Carrying a heavy purse, backpacks, or bags
- Chronic high heel use
- Driving too much
- Poor posture working on a computer
- Texting with your thumb
- Too much time sitting at your desk
- Wearing the wrong shoes

Sleeping
- Being a stomach sleeper
- Lack of quality sleep
- Sleeping on an old mattress

18 HABIT SHIFTING

"We have met the enemy and he is us"

—Walt Kelly

The phrase "We have met the enemy and he is us" first appeared on a poster to promote Earth Day in 1970. The creator, Walt Kelly, is also the creator of the Pogo comic strip and later used the phrase in a Pogo comic strip.

Introduction to Habit Shifting

Bad habits waste your energy. Yoga calls this your prana or life force. Bad habits keep you from accomplishing goals and from fully living your life. They can have negative effects on your physical and mental health. You struggle to find freedom from bad habits. When you break a bad habit, you often replace it with a different habit. It is easier to make changes if you focus on the benefits rather than point out a fault that needs correcting. You will practice two effective strategies to break a habit regardless of the habit you are trying to break.

The first strategy to break a bad habit is "learning to unlearn". The world will always continue to change and to survive you also must change. To succeed in life you must continue to learn, unlearn and relearn. You spend most of your time learning such as going to school. Rather than trying to learn a way to overcome an existing bad habit or behavior, try focusing on "unlearning" the behavior to make room for a positive one.

Before you can unlearn a habit, you should first understand the root cause. Bad habits can be a way of dealing with stress or boredom. Habits like biting your nails, overspending on a shopping spree, drinking every weekend or wasting time on the internet are often a response to stress and boredom. Sometimes you create the stress or boredom on the surface from having deeper issues. Working with these issues can be difficult and uncomfortable. If you are serious about making changes, you must push past the discomfort and change your habits and misbeliefs.

Remember you rarely remove a habit you replace it. Thinking about habits in this way can help you remove bad habits. Perhaps, instead of telling yourself "When I get stressed I need to stop biting my nails" try "When I get stressed I practice a breathing exercise".

The second strategy is to keep from giving up too early. Unlearning and relearning takes extra time and work. This will force you to change parts of your life and the people in it. Studies have shown that to create or break a habit you must practice a behavior for 28-40 days. After 28-40 days, it should become much easier. Have you noticed many diets are "30 day" miracle cures and fitness studios have low priced 30-day trials?

Remember, that failing is how you learn. Stay mindful that change is difficult and look for ways that will keep you accountable. Cut out as many triggers as possible. If you smoke when you drink, then stay out of bars. If you do not want to eat as many sweets do not keep buying them. Breaking a habit is much easier if you can avoid the things that cause them. Change your environment to make it easier to change bad habits. It also makes it easier to create new good habits.

Breaking bad habits takes time and effort with persistence being the most important part. Most people who break bad habits fail multiple times before they succeed. If you do not have immediate success, stay patient and you should see positive results.

Benefits of Positive Habits

"We are what we repeatedly do. Excellence then is not an act but a habit."

—Aristotle

A habit is a behavior pattern you often follow until it becomes almost involuntary. More than 40 percent of your actions are habits. Your brain does not know the difference between good habits and bad habits. You have to make that decision.

Habits can be extremely powerful tools for your personal growth and success. A positive habit is a positive action or behavior that produces positive benefits, attitudes, and actions. A healthy habit is a behavior that benefits your physical, emotional, and mental health.

Benefits of Positive Habits

- Better choices
- Boosts energy
- Combats diseases
- Controls weight
- Enhance outcomes
- Happier relationships
- Healthful lifestyle
- Help you reach your goals
- Higher spiritual connection
- Improves longevity
- Improves mood
- Increase competence
- More energy
- Perform more efficiently
- Promote comfort
- Saves time
- Sharpening focus
- Steadfast confidence
- Stronger foundation for life

Habit Shifting

In this two-part exercise on habits, you will identify a habit you wish to change. Then you will learn steps to create a new habit. The habits do not need to be similar.

Exercise 18.1 - Shift a Bad Habit

Stop a Bad Habit	Identify habit specifics.	Example:
1 Identify a habit you want to change.		• I have a sugar addiction.
2 How often do you do your habit? (Per day, week or month)		• 5-6 times a days
3 Where are you when the bad habit happens?		• I am at work.
4 Who are you with when your habit happens?		• I am by myself at my desk.

5		
What triggers the behavior and causes it to start?		• I need an energy and mood lift.
6 Identify a good behavior or "habit" you can use to replace the bad habit.		• I can eat a piece of fresh fruit, I can practice a breathing exercise quietly, or I can go for a short walk.
7 Identify ways to avoid situations and people that trigger your habit.		• I cannot avoid working alone at my desk. What I can do is to focus on work that requires another person either face-to-face or over the phone so I will not be alone.
8 Are there any other strategies you can use over the next 30 days to reinforce this change in your behavior? Remember that failure is a part of the learning process.		• I can bring cut up vegetables to work. I can also bring frozen grapes and take time to suck on them before eating.

Exercise 18.2 - Create a Positive Habit

Exercise Create a Positive Habit	Create your response.	Example:
1 Identify a positive habit you would like to create.		• I want to exercise more often.
2 How often do you want to do this habit? (Per day, week or month)		• I want to exercise three times a week.
3 What has prevented you from doing this?		• I lack time and energy after work to exercise.
4 What inspired you to make this change?		• I want to live pain free, feel better about my appearance, and enjoy the health benefits.

5 Identify a bad behavior or "habit" you need to stop.		• I will watch less television after work on days I exercise so I will have time to spend with my family and friends.
6 Identify a way to create a "trigger" situation and people who can help reinforce your new habit.		• I can find a friend to go to the gym with me and keep me accountable. •
7 Identify a way to avoid "trigger" situations and/or people who can help reinforce your new habit		• I can write a note on my mirror or create a vision board to remind myself of what inspires me to exercise.
8 Are there any other strategies you can use over the next 30 days to reinforce this change in your behavior? Remember that failure is a part of the learning process.		• I can sign up for yoga and exercise newsletters or podcasts to remind myself of the benefits of exercise. • I can write down three benefits I get from exercise and keep it in the top drawer of my desk as a reminder.

19 FEEL THE WAY YOU WANT TO FEEL

Life is better when you are laughing.

This chapter is adapted from a chapter in the book *Yoga Secrets: 52 Life-Changing Secrets*. It is difficult to find happiness when you are not living in the present moment. You view the past as better than it was, the present worse, and the future as hope and salvation. Your biggest threats to happiness are pain and boredom. To find your happiness, stay in the present by treating this moment as your first choice, regardless of the circumstances.

The Smiling Yoga Superpower

Smile as often as you can. Have you noticed that statues of the meditating Buddha show a half-smile on his face? A smile can quickly relax your mind, body, spirit, and even your physical pain.

Do What You Love

Mantra: "I will enjoy every moment of my journey."

Do what you love and learn to love what you have to do. Yoga helps you during your journey, and that is where you will find happiness. Happiness occurs when you totally focus on your quest. When you focus on your quest, time will pass as if it does not exist. Your concentration on your quest has distracted and freed you from depression, worries, and physical pain.

It is a common belief to search for happiness by climbing to the top of a mountain or to achieve something that is difficult. Lasting happiness is not at the top of a mountain or at the end of an accomplishment. Yoga helps you with your journey through life. You need to find happiness during your journey. Discover what you love and use your passion to go after it.

Acceptance

Mantra: "I will accept things as they happen."

Accept it, change it, or leave it. Accept things as they happen and treat the present moment as your first choice, regardless of the circumstances. To find happiness, stop over thinking everything in your life. Focusing on an event strengthens your attachment to that event. Your reluctance to detach from events comes from the misbelief in your life.

Practice learning, unlearning, and relearning. This should make it easier for you to change your habits and peel away your layers of misbelief.

Where Happiness Lies

Mantra: "I will laugh and smile with every breath."

Learn to love what you have to do. Laugh and smile as often as you can. Happiness is your natural state and happens when you stop making yourself unhappy. To stop making yourself unhappy, you need to keep your habits and misbelief from deciding how you make choices. Find freedom from habits and misbelief and choose your own path.

You need to train your mind for happiness. The more you practice being happy, the happier you will become. When I tell my students to give every living creature a smile, they respond by looking concerned that I am losing my mind. They are sure their smile will not help those other living creatures. They are learning a new way of seeing.

Act Happy To Be Happy

Mantra: "I will act happy to be happy."

Laugh and smile with every breath. It is easy to feel happy. You can feel the way you want to feel; just act the way you want to feel. To be energetic, act energetic. To be happy, act happy. Let go of your judgment and expectations. Start by pretending you are happy. How you act determines how you feel. Acting happy is easier if you stay mindful, practice nonreaction, and focus on how you want to feel.

Your brain is a muscle, and you need to train it to find happiness. Try smiling at every living creature you meet. For even more fun, give every living creature a half-smile or a fake smile. Have fun with it. This may sound too simple, but unlearn what you know and relearn it. It may surprise you how well this works.

Find More Happiness

- Act confident
- Be energetic
- Be enthusiastic
- Encourage curiosity
- Exercise
- Help someone
- Learn something new
- Practice gratitude
- Read something
- Smile
- Stop comparing
- Text a friend
- Think positive
- Try something new

20 MINDFULNESS

The only time that exists is the present moment.

The present moment is the only time when you have power and control. Fear pulls you back from the present moment, and desire pushes you past it. Both distract you from enjoying and living your life in the here and now.

Mindfulness is a practice that is thousands of years old. It requires you to stay active and pay attention, without judgment or attachment, to what is happening around you. You must carefully observe and accept your emotions, feelings, and thoughts. You stay in the present moment and thereby keep the world from passing you by. Mindfulness can calm your pain and assist you in acing your daily challenges. When you are in the present moment, it feels as if time ceases to exist, and it provides an escape from attachment to your problems.

To be mindful, you must purposefully observe what is happening around you. This creates clarity in your thoughts and in your life. Treat the present moment as your first choice, regardless of the circumstances. Experience and respond to things happening now. Stay present to cut back your anxiety. Mindfulness can help you find a new way of seeing things.

Practicing Mindfulness

To practice mindfulness, you must stop racing around and focus on what you are doing. Develop a habit of steady and calm breathing. This will slow your heart rate, calm your emotions, ease your mind, relax your muscles, and soften your body. Focus on inhaling and exhaling; start your inhale only as you completely finish your exhale. Breathe out what you do not want and breathe in gratitude and happiness.

Many important events in your life occur when you are not in the present, and you miss out on more important events and opportunities than you realize. Do not live as if you are not here. Your life will become easier, and you will find more energy and create more happiness in your life. Living in the past or the future keeps you from living in the present. It causes you to go through life as if you have never really lived.

Most of you find it difficult to stay mindful and in the present. It is natural to worry about the future or spend too much time dwelling on the past, but there is a time and place for everything, including reflecting on past actions and planning for future success. The exercise allows you to focus on the present moment, the only time when you truly have power and control. Explore three areas that keep you from being mindful and practice activities to overcome these obstacles.

First, you will cover habits, learning to unlearn, and developing persistence. Your habits often cause you to live on autopilot and prevent you from living in the present moment. Learning to identify bad habits and replace them with good habits can help you find freedom from the world that aims to control you through your emotions. This can help you calm your pain, stay mindful, and in the present moment. Creating positive habits, correcting misbeliefs, and letting go of things you cannot control will free up your prana, your life force, for more important things. Remember to accept where you are today. Make the easy changes first, and the harder ones will become easier. Always keep an open heart and mind.

Ways to Practice Mindfulness

Ask Better Questions
- Why are you here?
- What are your assumptions and beliefs, and why do you have them?
- What are your habits, and why do you have them?
- What are your thoughts, and why do you have them?

Attitude
- Be determined and follow your passion
- Learn to focus

Connect
- Connect with nature
- Connect with the present moment
- Connect with your senses

Disconnect
- Put your phone in airplane mode when in meetings
- Turn off your phone for several hours

Gratitude
- Tell someone how much you appreciate them
- Write a personal thank-you or love note

Non-reaction
- Observe your thoughts without attachment
- Observe your thoughts without reacting
- Practice acceptance
- Remain patient

Nourish
- Drink water all day
- Eat fresh, whole foods
- Eat slowly and savor every bite

Observe
- Observe your breathing
- Observe your emotions
- Observe your thoughts

Practice
- Practice steady, calm breathing
- Practice deep breathing
- Practice mindfulness
- Practice transformational listening

Simplify
- Act slowly and deliberately
- Do one thing at a time
- Eliminate distractions
- Eliminate the unimportant
- Slow down

Take Action
- Move around and stretch often
- Take short mindfulness breaks
- Use reminders, written and visual
- Write down your top three priorities every morning

Benefits of Mindfulness

Lowers
- Anxiety
- Blood pressure
- Depression
- Heart rate

Healthier
- Mind and body
- Social life and relationships

Increased
- Awareness, attention, and focus
- Clarity in thinking and perception
- Feeling of calmness, stillness, and openness
- Feeling of gratitude
- Immune function
- Path to insight
- Resilient mind
- Spiritual growth

PERSONAL SUMMARY

Question	Your Response
1 Which parts were most meaningful?	
2 Which parts were least meaningful?	
3 Which exercise(s) do you think will work best for creating change in your life?	
4 Do you plan to share any of the strategies and exercises with others? If so, which ones and with whom?	
5 Did you discover an area, habit, or belief that you would like to change in your life?	

ABOUT THE AUTHOR

Ken is a yoga author who trains yoga teachers how to add yoga philosophy to their classes to improve the lives of their students. His first book, *Yoga Secrets: 52 Life-Changing Secrets* published in 2016. It is among the first books written focused on teaching yoga philosophy during any style of yoga practice. He created a method to make it easy and fun for yoga teachers and for students. The book follows the Eight Limbs of Yoga from the Yoga Sutras of Patanjali. He is the founder of the GoalYoga™ Yoga Teacher Training School.

His practice of yoga spans over two decades. To fill your life with joy he believes you must have fun and humor in your yoga classes. His classes include life-changing lessons, fun, and silly jokes.

In early childhood, Ken asked questions that others thought were just odd. When he started his yoga practice, he asked many questions. He wanted to know the meaning of the terms and phrases he heard in class. This lead Ken to create the term "placebo phrase". Years later when teaching yoga he felt he needed to explain these "placebo phrases" to his students. He found this much harder than he had expected, which lead to creating Yoga Secrets.

Ken changed his career from focusing on things to focusing on people. He was managing and growing a national technology company he co-founded 30 years earlier. He taught yoga and created lessons as often as he could.

While teaching a lesson for students to ask better questions, he asked one of himself. What should he do next? This was an easy answer and a much harder transition. He wanted to share his fun and easy method of transforming people's lives. Knowing what you want to do and actually doing it are very different. He knew those in his groups or tribes would not approve of this change. It took time for him to realize he was not in search of their approval, he was in search of his true self. He made the change.

Ken had adopted the beliefs of others that yoga was not something you did as a career, it was something you did for exercise and fun. He had to unlearn this belief and relearn a new belief. This sounds easy to do when giving advice, but very challenging when you are the one who is changing. He found help by using the lessons from yoga he was creating for his students.

He has tested and refined this method and these lessons in thousands of yoga classes. This simple method uses specific techniques to help make changes and to have them last. Several of the techniques include persistence, clarity, learning to unlearn, and frequency versus duration.

After changing his career, Ken trained yoga teachers and wrote *Yoga Secrets*. His passion is to share the life-changing lessons of yoga to help anyone who wants to change their life.

He knows his students practicing their yoga postures will get better balance, focus, discipline, and strength. However, will their life be better? Will they strive for the miraculous?

Ken always lived with a fear of writing. He could write boring and polite business communication. When he tried to go further, it would swell his level of anxiety. While writing *Yoga Secrets* he was in constant fear and anxiety of not being able to write the book. His motivation was the pain of not sharing the lessons would be much greater than the pain of writing the book. He used the lessons in *Yoga Secrets* to overcome his anxiety of writing.

He has a background in fitness and health. Before yoga, Ken taught aerobic classes, ran marathons, and backpacked. He has a Bachelor of Science in Food Science and Nutrition from North Carolina State University and an MBA in Information Systems from Golden Gate University.

Ken Heptig